MW01293103

MED MATH SIMPLIFIED

Dosing Math Tricks for Students, Nurses, and Paramedics

Jamie Davis, RN, NRP, BA

First edition published Dec 2014
Copyright © 2014 MedicCast Productions, LLC

DEDICATED TO

Amy, Saralynn, Mindy, and Chris
   Thanks for putting up with me and my various ventures!

FOREWARD

Hi, I'm Jamie Davis, the Podmedic, host of popular online radio programs such as <u>The Nursing Show</u> (<u>NursingShow.com</u>) and the <u>MedicCast Podcast</u> (<u>MedicCast.com/blog</u>). I wanted to personally welcome you to this book on medication math. I think that this an important topic for all of us to review from time to time.

You have purchased this book because you are struggling with successfully computing medication math problems. I want you to know you are not alone. I like to consider myself a pretty bright guy but when it comes to math I really struggle. I know there are people who just get math. It comes easy to them. In fact, I married one of them.

Let me tell you a story about my math struggles. Maybe it will be familiar to you. When going to nursing school, I had to take a pre-calculus course as part of my degree program. It was far and above the hardest course I took and I would spend hours pouring over the homework to make sure I got it figured out. I could do the work but I really had to plod along to get it right.

One night I was sitting at the kitchen table after dinner with my textbook open and a pile of paper and scrap paper piled around me. I had been struggling with the same problem for at least an hour and just couldn't get it. My wife walked by me. She majored in math in college and always said that calculus was one of her favorite courses. She looked over my shoulder and said, "Oh, I remember doing that." She grabbed a sheet of paper and a pencil and proceeded to work the problem. In about five minutes, she was done. "That was fun!" she said. Then she walked away, taking the solution to the problem with her.

Something like this might have happened to you. Maybe it was a friend, a spouse, or a classmate. It is frustrating. Frankly, for a lot of us, math is just frustrating and that includes drug calculations. Whether you are a nurse, physician, paramedic, or other medical professional, medication and drug calculations are a necessary part of your job. Patient safety depends on you calculating correctly each and every time.

This book, the website at MedMathSimplified.com/ebook and accompanying materials are all designed by me, a math idiot, to review and refresh medication math for medical professionals at all levels. We'll take the basic concepts and break them down, simplifying them for you (and me). The goal is to make you a better health care professional, provide better and safer patient care, and ultimately give you more time to do what you do best, care for your patients. This is Med Math Simplified.

MATH PHOBIA?

Does math drive you nuts?

Does it take you what seems like hours to complete your calculations?

ME, TOO!

I know that a lot of people who listen to my shows online think I'm some kind of genius paramedic or nurse to do what I do. No, I work hard to produce the materials, research the facts, and when it comes to math, I fall back on tried and true techniques to make it easier for me.

Still think you can't do it?

I think you can and I'll tell you why . . .

If you can learn and master the steps of a basic patient assessment, learn to apply your skills to take care of your patient, whether in the hospital or on an ambulance, then I am confident that you can learn the methodical steps to become a confident medical mathematician!

That's right! You can be a Medical Mathematician. There is no secret to this. The typical math that is used to correctly figure doses and patient weight conversions and IV drip rates are all based on just a few basic formulas.

Learn to construct those formulas correctly and plug in the values correctly and the rest is just addition, subtraction, multiplication and division. So ultimately, all you need to do this is the math you learned in elementary school.

The problem with most students whom I've met is they look at math and their eyes cross. Seriously! It's as if everything starts to swim around and before they know it everything just becomes a big jumble of numbers and signs. If only they had a step by step plan, a way of doing things that would allow them to be successful and safe when calculating patient doses and other medical math (like metric conversions).

This program is going to be a road map to success for you. No one goes on a trip to a destination by just randomly driving and expecting to get there, or at least get there in a reasonable time frame. You have to plan your trip, make a map of your destinations and make reservations for the places you want to stay. Getting to the right dose for your patients is no different. You have to make a plan to get there successfully each time, every time. You DO NOT want to be arriving at medication dosages by accident!

Since accidental dosing is not a desired patient outcome, we need to come up with a better way, together, to get the job done. Here's what we're going to do. We're going to take things step by step - plan our approach so that every calculation becomes the same. We will follow the same steps and complete the problem, the same way, every time. We'll start out with a review of some basic math and algebra concepts and common conversions needed for medical calculations. Then we will get into the

Med Math Simplified plan for every formula. Finally, we'll touch on some of the tricks and short cuts that are out there and why it's not a good idea to become too reliant on them all of the time.

How to Use This Book

I wrote this book as a guide to people with math skills at all levels. Some of you have just a basis in high school math while others are in college or beyond. As you read this book you may encounter math skills reviewed that you already possess. Great, that is awesome news. I urge you, however, to avoid skipping past sections because you think you know what is inside or how to do the math in those chapters. At least skim the material and mentally review the calculations as you go through the book. This program for medication math is built on a series or steps or building blocks. Don't skip a step. You might end up missing an important part of a formula later in the book because you didn't review something earlier in the book.

Also, take the practice quizzes and exercises at the end of the book (there are more at MedMathSimplified.com/ebook). Take the time to work through them. These are in place to help you be more successful later on. They help you have success early on so that you are not overwhelmed later when you get to more complex problems. You might be able to convert metric system measurements like converting pounds to kilograms in your head because you've been doing it for patients for a long time. Take the time to do those metric conversion problems in the book and make sure you have truly mastered it without using a trick or conversion you have already memorized.

Who is This Book For?

You might be wondering if this book is for you. Well

that is a perfectly good question to ask so let's set the stage for who might best benefit from this book. This ebook is a good fit for students in a variety of health careers. Student nurses (RN and LPN), paramedics, emergency medical technicians, pharmacists, even medical students might benefit from a brief refresher included in this book.

The question you need to ask is to determine which part you might play if you acted out that story I told earlier. You know the one about my own math struggles and the experience with my wife quickly writing out a problem? If you feel like you could play the part of my wife then this book might not be for you. Your confidence in your math abilities is obviously stronger than mine. Go for it! You don't need this book to do your medication math dosing safely.

If, however, you think you might best be cast in the role I played in that story. If you are the person who struggles with getting math problems set up correctly and who gets frustrated or anxious when working through math problems then this book might be good for you. If you are the type of person who might fail out of their health career program in college because you cannot do the required medication math pretest each semester then this book is good for you.

Perhaps you are a nurse, paramedic or other health professional already working in the field of your choice but think you might need a refresher for an upcoming class like Advanced Cardiac Life Support (ACLS) or Pediatric Advanced Life Support (PALS). Your ability to complete these courses or refresh them often relies on correct medication dosing and the ability to do so quickly and confidently. If you are prepping for one of those courses then you might be a person who needs this particular book.

Maybe you are considering a career in the healthcare field and want to know if you have the math skills to do the work with patients and medication dosing? This book would be an excellent check of your current mathematics skills in the particular area of medication dosing math. You could work through this book and find out what additional areas you need to work through in your preparation for formal course work. Whatever your concerns about doing safe and correct medication math, this book and collection of exercises is the one for you.

Ok, it is time to get started on your Med Math Simplified journey. By the end of this book, it is my hope that you will be ready to conquer all your medication math problems with confidence but if you still need more help there is an additional nine part video companion series you may purchase that goes with this book. It walks you through the problems again for those of you that are visual learners. It will help you be more successful at med math. You can find that at MedMathSimplified.com/ebook.

ON SAFETY AND MEDICATIONS

Before we get started we should take a few moments to talk about safety and medication dosing. There are some important concepts we must review about how to safely note medications and doses. The correct notation of doses for medications is of utmost importance. For most of you this will be a review of basic medication safety but I urge you not to skip over it. This is a short but very important section of this book. Read through it and refresh your commitment to the **"Five Rs of Medication Safety."**

What are the "Five Rs" or "Five Rights of Medication Safety" you ask? These are the things that you must ask yourself before giving any patient any medication. One of them is the reason for this book. It is simply "Right Dose." But there are other, equally important rights for medication administration and safety that are just as important and go hand in hand with "Right Dose." The Five Rights are:

- Right Medication
- Right Expiration Date
- Right Patient

- Right Route of Administration
- Right Dose

Let's look at each of the Five Rights in turn to make sure we understand all of them.

Right medication is the first and it seems kind of simple-minded to some. However the Institute for Safe Medication Practices (ISMP.org) has a list 9 pages long of commonly confused medications. These are medications that have names that are similar sounding when spoken aloud or similar looking when written out. If you want to see some of them for yourself visit the ISMP site for the complete list. You must compare the medication you are preparing to administer to the medication ordered and make sure it is the same.

Right expiration date is next up in the Five Rights and it, too seems simple. Often however, we don't check expiration dates on medications we administer. We might assume that someone else has rotated the medication stocks to make sure that we use the oldest medication first and thus use meds before they expire. For infrequently used medications that sit in a drawer or on a shelf, however, that may not be the case. How do you know if you don't check? It is a best practice to review the dates of any medication as a matter of routine so that you always catch out of date medications when they pop up.

Right patient is a very important step. In a hospital setting where you might be caring for many patients, it is easy to get your orders mixed up. You should verify that you have the right patient by checking their ID bracelet with their written orders to make sure you have the correct one. Even in a setting like home health care or in the back of an ambulance, checking some patient facts is important. While you may only have one patient at a time there are things about some medications that make it important to confirm they are the right patient for the drug at hand. Some drugs are not recommended for pregnant women for example. Some patients are allergic to some medications. Confirm they have no allergies to the medication at hand before you continue. Make sure they are the right patient for the drug.

Right route of administration is next and is equally important. How is the drug you are preparing to administer supposed to be introduced into the body? You must understand the differences between the various routes of administration. Some methods are more slowly absorbed than others. Your job is to know the correct routes of administration for the medications you are giving and know which of those routes is the most appropriate for a given situation.

Right Dose comes last and, as I have already said, that is the primary purpose of this book. We must be able to calculate the correct dose for each patient. There is more to dose than that, though. How you write that dose out for others to read back is also important. There are very specific rules surrounding how to write out medication doses correctly so that mistakes in dosing are avoided. When writing the doses out in your calculations, you must avoid writing the dose in such a way that someone else might make an error when reading it back or in the patient's chart.

No Trailing Zeros - Look at the following dose for epinephrine 1:10,000 in cardiac arrest. Are you to administer 1.0 milligram (mg) or are you to administer 1 milligram (mg)? Which is correct? The second one is the correct answer. The first is too easy to mistake for 10 (ten) milligrams of epinephrine because the decimal point might be missed when reading it. The rule is no trailing zeros are to be used when writing a medication dose.

Use Leading Zeros - Similarly, look at the following dose for epinephrine 1:1,000 in cases of allergic reaction. Are you to administer 0.5 milligrams (mg) or are you to administer .5 milligrams (mg)? Which is correct? In this case the first answer is the correct one. Again, you might miss the decimal point in the second choice and administer 5 mg by mistake, a definite harmful mistake for the patient. The rule is to use a leading zero before the decimal point to draw attention to it and make sure that the correct dose is given.

Now that we've looked at some medication safety issues and reviewed the Five Rights, it is time to move on in the book. Next up we will look at some math basics to make sure we are all on the same page moving forward. In the next chapter, there will be some links to additional resources to do basic math review to make sure you are ready for the rest of the book.

MATH BASICS

To get started we need to review some basic mathematics. I will assume you have the necessary skills to do basic addition, subtraction, multiplication and division. If you need some help with these mathematical operations, it is no big deal. We will not cover it here but there are plenty of resources out there for you to use. Try these websites to review your basic math skills and then come back here and continue on with the Med Math Simplified steps.

Online Math Resources
http://www.math.com/students/practice.html
http://www.purplemath.com
http://www.sosmath.com
http://www.mathsisfun.com

Use the resources above and plenty of others you can search for on Google to get you started on the basics.

Getting Started - Order of Operations
The first thing we need to cover is that some things in math have to happen in a certain order. When completing a difficult math problem like the one below you have to do things in a certain order. This is called the order of

operations.

$$6(9+3-7)/2=?$$

What do you start with in this problem? If you do not pick the right starting point, the answer will be wrong and you know that. The most common way of remembering this is the one I learned back in elementary school. It is PEMDAS. The way to remember this is to remember the mnemonic sentence - "Please Excuse My Dear Aunt Sally." I don't know who Aunt Sally is or what she was continuously doing that required forgiveness, but this is how many of us learned to do the order of operations. It stands for "Parentheses, Exponents, Multiplication, Division, Addition, Subtraction."

That is the order of operations. In the problem above you first work the math inside the parenthesis, addition first, then subtraction. So, in this case, the parenthesis shows a problem to solve within the larger problem. Using the PEMDAS formula inside the parenthesis we find first that nine plus three is twelve. Then we do the next part in the PEMDAS order and find that twelve minus seven is five. Now the problem looks like this:

$$6(5)/2=?$$

Now we use PEMDAS to finish the problem. Multiplication goes first with six times five equaling thirty. Next we do the division and get thirty divided by two to equal fifteen. So the answer to the original problem is fifteen.

$$6(9+3-7)/2=15$$

Let's try another one together, ok? We will do a few problems together and get through them until we are confident on this.

$$4+2*3=?$$

This problem is pretty straight forward. PEMDAS tells us to go through and do the multiplication first. Two times three equals six. Next we do the addition to get four plus six equals ten. So this solution is:

$$4+2*3=10$$

Let's try a more complex one this time. Don't get discouraged if it looks to busy for you. Take Aunt Sally's formula and do it one step at a time.

$$4+(2+1)^2=?$$

Take PEMDAS and do it one step at a time. Start with the items in the parenthesis and execute the addition there. Two plus one is three. So now the problem looks like this:

$$4+(3)^2=?$$

Now using PEMDAS we will take care of the exponent. The superscript two there on the problem means to square the number in the parenthesis or multiply it by itself. That means that it is a multiplication problem. Three times three is nine. Now the problem says:

$$4+9=?$$

* * *

Finally we end up with a simple addition problem. Four plus nine is thirteen, leaving us with the answer:
$$4+9=13$$

That is the way to work through a problem. Take it step by step using the simple skills you come up with along the way like Aunt Sally's formula, PEMDAS. We will be working through complex problems by turning them into a series of simple problems. One step at a time. That is how the Med Math Simplified system works.

Cross Cancelation

The next basic algebra skill is solving equations where there are complex formulas with values on top and bottom of an equation where some of them are the same. For instance, look at the common med math problem below. This is one of the problems we will look at periodically through the book as we learn to layout the formulas correctly. In this case, though we will just look at how the concept of cross cancelation works.

$$\frac{?\,gtts}{minutes} = \frac{60\,gtts}{1mL} * \frac{250mL}{400mg} * \frac{5mcg}{minute} * \frac{1mg}{1000m\varepsilon}$$

When laying out a problem like this, we can get rid of a lot of the extraneous values by canceling items that appear in the top and bottom (and on the same side) of the equation. This is what that would look like in this case:

$$\frac{?\,gtts}{minutes} = \frac{60\,gtts}{1} * \frac{250}{400} * \frac{5}{minute} * \frac{1}{1000}$$

Look at the example above and see how it works. For

every value that is the same in the numerator (top) or denominator (bottom) we can cancel them out. So we were able to cancel out the micrograms value (mcg), the milligrams value (mg), the milliliters value (mL) leaving the much simpler problem listed below:

$$\frac{?\,gtts}{minutes} = \frac{75,000\,gtts}{400,000\,minutes}$$

This is just a math problem now. We can work the multiplication and come up with the partial solution. We can now get rid of some of those zeros, too. Just use the cancelation method again.

$$\frac{?\,gtts}{minutes} = \frac{75\,gtts}{400\,minutes}$$

Do the math to get the answer of:

$$\frac{?\,gtts}{minutes} = \frac{1\,gtts}{5.33\,minutes}$$

Now you might think this makes no sense but it is part of a larger equation where we calculate a rate for a patient of a certain weight in kilograms. The real equation is going to be:

$$\frac{?\,gtts}{minutes} = \frac{1\,gtts\,/\,kg}{5.33\,minutes}$$

But solving this would be easy, right? Your 75 kilogram patient is going to get a drug delivered at 75 drops (gtts) per 5.33 minutes using a micro drip IV setup. Do the math and you end up with a drip rate of 14.07 or just 14 drops per minute.

Bookmark this section of the book. You might need to come back to it. We'll be using the strategies and lessons here all through the Med Math Simplified series to work through the problems later in the book.

THE METRIC SYSTEM!!!!

Now let us look at the metric system, the most confusing, odd form of measurement known to man. Ok, maybe that's a bit much. Actually, for the rest of the world, our standard of measurement here in the U.S. in inches, feet, ounces and pounds is just as confusing. For some of you, this metric system overview may be an easy review. For others, this may be the basis of your med math challenges. The important part is to stick around and review this info together so we can move forward. This is the basis of everything that follows.

The Metric system is actually pretty easy when you stop and look at it objectively. It is entirely based on units of ten. If you can count by tens and hundreds then the numbers are easy in the metric system. I have found, though, that the base units and prefixes tend to mix people up so we'll spend most of our time focusing on those. Just remember that the next higher or lower units of measure are either bigger or smaller by a factor of 10. Simply add or remove a zero, or move a decimal point left or right to convert the number to the next smaller or larger unit of measure.

Metric base units:

- **Meter** is a unit of length or in really big lengths - distance. If you measure a pencil, it is a simple length measurement but measure how far it is to the next town, and it is better thought of as a distance. Still, it all is based on the meter as the root term. A Meter is roughly equivalent to a yard in english measure or 3 feet. For reference, a average man is just under 2 meters tall.

- **Gram** is a unit of weight or mass. Depending on the thing being measured, it will either be a really big number (something heavy) or small number (lightweight). A gram is about the weight of paper clip. So it is pretty small.

- A **Liter** is a unit of volume or displacement. It is roughly equal to a quart in English measure.

- **Centigrade** or **Celsius** is the metric standard of measurement for temperature. It is based on the freezing and boiling point for water at sea level. Freezing is 0 degrees Celsius. Boiling is 100 degrees Celsius. Normal body temperature is 37 degrees Celsius.

Ok, so now you have mastered the base units of measurement in the metric system. Now let's move on to the metric prefixes. Remember each is a multiple of 10's so you are just adding or subtracting zeroes, or moving the decimal a certain number of places to the right or left.

Common Metric Prefixes:

- **Kilo** is the largest measure we'll see in patient care - You will most commonly see this in measures of weight where you are estimating a patient's weight or converting from pounds to <u>KILOgrams</u>. Kilo signifies one thousand times the base unit so a Kilogram is one thousand grams. Similarly, a kilometer is one thousand meters. There is even a kiloliter although it is not commonly used.

> •   Next in commonly seen prefixes we move smaller with **Centi** which reduces the base unit by 100. You will most commonly see this is describing wounds or short distances on a body: for instance, the wound was 2 cm across and was 5 cm to the left of the patient's midline. A centimeter is 1/100 of a meter. You will most likely only use this in terms of length or distance and not for weights or volume.

> •   Next on our list is **Milli**. This makes the base unit one thousand times smaller. It is going to be the most commonly seen prefix in medication math as it refers to really small divisors of the base units. For instance 1 mg is 1/1,000 of a gram (that's 1/1,000 of that paperclip mentioned earlier). This is useful for volume measurement as well, since a liter is so large, a milliliter (mL) is a much easier unit of measurement for dosing medications in solutions.

> •   Finally, **Micro**. This reduces the base unit one million times and will most commonly be used in weights in micrograms. This is really small but it is important to note the difference and be very careful. If you mistake a microgram measurement for a milligram measurement, you will give the patient one thousand time their normal dose so be careful!

Common Metric Abbreviations

We have looked over the metric standards of measurement for length, volume and mass. We have also covered the common metric prefixes. For the rest of this book, and in your travels in healthcare, there are common abbreviations for these units of measure with their prefixes and root words. You must learn to recognize them and to learn which ones are at risk of being confused with others in order to safely deliver medication to a patient.

- **milligram** = mg
- **microgram** = m c g o r sometimes ug (u signifying Greek letter mu)
- **milliliter** = mL or sometimes ml

A note about micrograms. The use of ug is falling out of favor because when handwritten quickly, the U can look like an M and might be mistaken for the abbreviation of milligrams (mg). Be careful and follow your institution's rules and guidelines for medication safety when documenting doses and metric abbreviations.

NON-STANDARD UNITS OF MEASURE

We have looked at the standard of measurement for science and medicine. Now we will look at non-standard units of measure including the old apothecary system. This system is being phased out but you may find an older physician who still prescribes using this system. The apothecary system is based in old, non-standardized weights and measures. This means that depending on your textbook or reference source, you might have two different conversions to milliliters from drams.

The Joint Commission guidelines for medication safety and error reduction would call this a violation of standard practices and I, personally, would not take an order written this way. In cases where I received an order written in non-standard units, I would ask the doctor to rewrite it or a pharmacist to convert it for me.

Here are some samples from the apothecary system:

- **dram** = ~ 4 mL
- **minim** = ~ .06 mL
- **grain** = ~ 60 mg

Other non-standard measurements include the one's

listed below. These are somewhat more important since they are more commonly needed in calculations. For instance, converting from pounds to kilograms happens quite frequently.

- **pounds** (lbs.) = .45 kg (2.2 lb/ kilogram)

- **teaspoon** (t.) = 5 mL
- **tablespoon** (T.) = 15 mL
- **ounce** = 30 mL

Conversions from teaspoons is useful for medications in solution for oral administration (pediatric meds particularly). A teaspoon is equivalent to 5 mL. The teaspoon is being phased out because a teaspoon is also the common name for a spoon in your flatware set. These sets of tableware are not standardized in any way. Dosing, therefore is better with a small measuring cup or special spoon or syringe designed for medications. The same is true of the tablespoon, since many unknowing parents may just use a bigger spoon like a soup spoon or serving spoon. A tablespoon is three teaspoons or 15 mL.

Dangers of Non-Standard Units of Measure

Recently recommended changes in dosing protocols for children's medications that are commonly formulated in liquid forms have come about. This is due to problems with dosing recommendations using non-standard units of measurement like teaspoons. There have been numerous reports of younger children being unintentionally overdosed on medications like acetaminophen because parents have used spoons like those intended for table settings as measurements for children's medication. Just because a spoon for table service is called a tea spoon (because it is used to stir tea or coffee) does not mean that it holds a teaspoon worth of liquid. Often it will hold more than a standard teaspoon, causing dosing problems for parents and children.

The American Academy of Pediatrics released the following statement on the practice of prescribing medications using non-standard measurements.

"Pediatricians [and other health care professionals] are encouraged to help prevent unintentional medication overdoses by eliminating the practice of prescribing medications with volumes in teaspoons and tablespoons. Instead, metric-based dosing using milliliters (mLs) for all liquid medicine prescriptions is preferred." AAP PROTECT Task Force Recommendation

Likewise, pharmacies are being encouraged to give out dosing spoons or syringes marked only in milliliters (mL). The hope is patients will only have those devices with which to measure medications for their children. The goal of this initiative is to significantly reduce the common errors in dosing that parents are unwittingly making through education and provision of the proper tools.

CONVERSION MATH FORMULAS

Now let us look at conversions we might use in the care of a patient. These will be conversions between metric measures as well as conversions between metric and the non-standard weights and measures. This requires setting up an equation that you will then solve with some basic math. Setting up these equations or formulas is the key to correctly figuring med math. The formula is the most important part of the process so let's look a basic version of the formula first.

Formula Layout:

        1.   Figure out which value you want (what is the test question asking you for?)

        2.   Place that requested value on the left side of the equation

        3.   Figure out the value(s) you have

        4.   Place that on the right side of the equation.

        5.   Determine your conversion values.

        6.   Multiply the value you have by

the conversion values.

Let's start with a basic conversion you will likely be running all of the time - converting pounds to kilograms. Here's the practice problem:

You have a patient who weighs 220 pounds. What is his weight in kilograms (kg)?

Yeah, I know. We can all do this one in our heads. It seems like for the purposes of most paramedic weight guesses, every adult male is exactly 100 kilos, and every adult female is exactly 50 kilos, right? Seriously, though, get in the habit of setting up these problems correctly from the start. Even on the easy ones.

Look at the question again and follow our steps in laying out the equation for the first time.

1. What do you want to know? The weight in kilograms.

2. Place it on the left side of the equals sign.

3. What do you know? The weight in pounds.

4. Place the weight in pounds on the right side of the equals sign.

5. What is the conversion? 2.2 pounds per kilograms.

6. Divide the weight in pounds by the conversion value 2.2 pounds per kilogram.

NOTE: As you build the formula you'll need to keep a few rules in mind. you want the value labels to cross cancel out as shown earlier in this book under the math review. Turn the conversion value around (upside down) when needed to match the equation set up.

In this case we will turn the 2.2 pounds per kilogram

over and say it's 1 kilogram per 2.2 pounds. You need to get in the habit of doing that to make sure you get the answers you want, the correct answer. Put the corresponding value you want on top on the opposite side of the equation.

$$?kg = 220pounds * \frac{1kg}{2.2pounds}$$

So let's convert this one. First, cancel out the pieces of the equation you can. Remember our review from earlier in this book on basic math and algebra? you may cancel values or like numbers on a one for one basis from the the top and bottom of the equation. That leaves you with 220 times one kilogram, divided by 2.2. Do the math and you get 100 kg.

$$?kg = 220 * \frac{1kg}{2.2}$$

Or

$$?kg = 100kg$$

Now, you've been saying the whole time I go through this, "Jamie, I already know that one. I can do it in my head!" and you are right. But this is about setting up the equation so that you can run the equation the same way, each and every time you need to do so.

Let's try one more. The bag of saline you have is labeled one Liter. How many milliliters do you have? I know you can do this in your head, too. Humor me and set up the equation anyway. You will thank me for the practice later, I swear!

Ok, let's set up the equation again.

1.   What do you want to know? How many milliliters do you have.

2.   What do you know? You have 1 Liter.

3.   What is the conversion you need to use here? 1 Liter is equal to 1,000 milliliters.

Setting up the problem we'll put the value we want on the left, the value we know on the right and multiply it by the conversions we need to use. See if your scrap paper matches what we have below.

$$?mL = 1 Liter * \frac{1000mL}{1 Liter}$$

Did you set it up right? Remember to flip values around so we can cross cancel items out. Ok, now we will cancel out the values we can and that leaves us with our answer because we do not have to do much math in this one.

$$?mL = 1 * \frac{1000mL}{1}$$

Or

$$?mL = 1000mL$$

Time to review some key points before we move on to laying out more complex equations.

• Understand the underlying relationships of the Metric system. Know the different factors of ten for each of the various prefixes and how they modify the base values up or down.

- Remember that non-standard conversions are out there even as we strive for a universal safe dosing and medication standard. It is important to recognize them and to memorize at least a few of them.
- Do the Math. The last part you have to do. Sorry, no tricks here. If you think you need additional resources or refresher here about basic math or algebra, I'd suggest talking to your school about what resources and tutoring they make available. Or go back to the math review website suggestions from the earlier chapter on Math Basics.

LAYING OUT THE FORMULAS

There are four parts to laying out your formulas correctly and they all have to do with gathering and ordering your information. When you are asked a question on a test or quiz, you are given a set of information. That information is what you will draw from to answer the question.

In some cases, there may be more information than you need and part of your job will involve weeding out the information that is important from the information that is not important. Setting up your formula correctly will help with that task but the weeding out process is part of another whole lesson on testing strategies that I am not going into at this time.

Gather your information starting with your orders or what your test question or your end dose for your patient is asking you. In the case of orders, that would be from your EMS protocols, hospital standing orders, or from an order from a prescriber such as a nurse practitioner or physician. It will be in a form such as "administer 20 mL/ kg fluid resuscitation." The structure of the value you need will often be in the form of a fraction or dose in milligrams per milliliter.

What Final Dose Do You Need?

- "mg/mL"
- "g/L"
- "Drops/minute (or gtts/min)"
- "mg/hour"
- "tablets/dose"

In the case of a test question, it is usually stated in clear terms although it may be inferred. For instance, look at this test question:

A doctor writes orders for a patient to receive 4 mg of morphine sulfate IV push PRN for complaints of sharp pain. You have a vial with 10 milligrams of morphine sulfate in 10 milliliters of normal saline solution in the vial.

There is no question specifically asked here but you would infer that an IV push indicates liquid measurement so you would use a syringe and the answer would be in milliliters. So, the question here is really asking "How many milliliters (mL) do we need?"

Next, after we have determined what our question or orders are asking us for, let's move on to looking at the available medications or concentration on hand. This may be a multiple step process in complex problems but we'll keep it to one step right now. You are looking for labeling information on your medication vials or IV bags such as:

- "mg/mL"
- "g/L"
- ". . . mg dissolved in . . ."
- "1 tablet contains . . ."

In our previous question, this would be 10 mg of morphine sulfate in 10 mL of normal saline.

Finally, look at the orders or test question and determine what conversions you need to be prepared to do. This might be converting patient weight from pounds to kilograms or another conversion. Remember to use your metric system knowledge from our conversions segment of this book. Factors of 10 are key as is memorizing the following frequently used conversions.

- 1 gram = 1,000 mg
- 1 mg = 1,000 mcg
- 1 L = 1,000 mL
- Drip Set Factor is # gtts/mL

Now that you've gathered your information let's layout out our pieces using the formula we looked at during the conversion review earlier. I can't stress enough that no matter how complex your problem is, if you lay it out this way and work through it methodically, you will be successful. It might even seem easy after a little practice.

Time and again, when I show this process to people, the mistakes are made when people try to cut corners. Take this step by step and don't skip steps because you think you can combine things and do the math in your head. That is where the mistakes happen. We'll look at a simple problem now and then tackle a more complex one later on.

Let's look at the medication math problem from the example earlier. Remember to gather information. It isn't a bad idea to write down the items as you come to them. Use plenty of scrap paper or if you need it, there will usually be room on the test page to write your work down as you move along.

Orders: Give patient 4 mg of morphine.

Medication on hand: You have a 10 mL vial with 10 mg

of morphine inside.

How many mL do you draw up? That is the problem from before.   Let's look at the information we have and start laying the problem out for you.

Start with what the problem is asking for and put it on the LEFT: How many mL?

On the right side start with Concentration on hand. It is very important to make sure that the value label (mL, mg, gtts, etc.) on the top (the numerator) is the same on both sides of the equation. 10 mL/10 mg

Fill in ordered dose to the right, in this case that is 4 mg ordered.

. I will not write this one out for you. You should have practiced this in the previous chapter. Refer back to that chapter and the one on math review if you need to. Remember that you can cancel values and numbers that are the same on the top as the bottom of the equation. If you have set your problem up correctly, you will alternate values top and bottom starting with the first items set up to the right until you have all information accounted for. When you cancel out, you are left with the values you need. In this problem, that is milliliters. Then you just do the math which in this situation is easy since the only number left is four! The correct answer to this problem is 4 mL to be drawn up into the syringe.

Ok, let's do a more complex problem this time. Now for those nurses in the hospital or transport paramedics with IV pumps, this dopamine problem doesn't crop up very often any more. The issue, however, is one that is faced by anyone without an IV pump, so we'll take it on. It is also a common question on many paramedic tests and exams. Let's read the problem together and then lay it out. First gather your information.

Orders: 5 mcg/kg/min Dopamine

You have a 250 mL bag with 400 mg of Dopamine inside and a 100 kg patient. How many drops per minute do you set using minidrip set (60 gtts/ml)?

This question is going to be more complex but don't cross your eyes and decide it's too hard. Complex does not mean hard. It just has a few more steps. The individual steps are all simple. So let's take it one step at a time. First, what is the problem or order asking for? What do you need to know at the end? In this case, to give the dopamine to this patient using a minidrip IV set (60 drops or gtts per mL), you need to know how many drops per minute to administer. Ok, place that on the left. Cool, step one done.

Next, we usually start with concentration on hand but since this question is asking for drip rate, let's use the drip set concentration information. The drip set is 60 drops per milliliter. This is important because we want to make sure our final values match from left to right. Match up the drops on the top and with mL on the bottom.

Now add in the drug we have on hand. Now we could call this 400 mg in 250 mL but we want to alternate values top and bottom. Since we already have mL on the bottom here with the drip rate, let's put mL on the top so we can cancel it out. This means we have 250 mL/400 mg. Next we add the ordered dose of 5 mcg/kg/minute. Since we have a weight measure (mg) on the bottom, let's put the micrograms on the top here. We can convert that to milligrams in a separate step or if you'd like we can next add in the value 1 mg/1,000 mcg.

You are doing this along with me, right? Ok, we need to

add in one more part, the weight of the patient is 100 kg so the final part is to add the value 100 kg to the equation. If you have laid out the problem correctly it should look something like this.

$$\frac{?\,gtts}{min} = \frac{60\,gtts}{1mL} * \frac{250mL}{400mg} * \frac{5mcg}{kg/min} * \frac{1mg}{1000mcg} *$$

Cancel out the values on top and bottom as you have learned.

$$\frac{?\,gtts}{min} = \frac{60\,gtts}{1} * \frac{250}{400} * \frac{5}{min} * \frac{1}{1000} * 100$$

Don't forget the zeros. You can cancel some of them out, too.

$$\frac{?\,gtts}{min} = \frac{6\,gtts}{1} * \frac{25}{4} * \frac{5}{min} * \frac{1}{10} * 1$$

Now do the math to get:

$$\frac{?\,gtts}{min} = \frac{750\,gtts}{40min}$$

Or

$$\frac{?\,gtts}{min} = \frac{18.75\,gtts}{min}$$

The answer you get is 18.75 drops per minute. Since we can't give a partial drop we will round that up to 19 drops per minute. If your eyes crossed a few times doing that problem, don't worry. That is about the most complex item you will have to do. If it seems too complex, look at it in parts. First convert the dose for the particular patient. Then convert micrograms per minute to milligrams per minute. This will shorten the final portion of the formula significantly.

Those are two examples to start you off. There are more materials in the video series and tutorial at MedMathSimplified.com/ebook. These include several practice quizzes with additional practice problems to work through with the answers to check your work. There are also more practice questions at the end of this book (with the answers).

Before we end this part, let's review:

REVIEW:

- Review Your Conversions
- Gather Information
- Layout Your Problem
- Run The Math
- Check Answer Against Knowledge

USING TABLES AND CHARTS

This section in the Med Math Simplified book is going to cover using tricks, short cuts and tables. We will start with using pre-made tables that you might find in a pocket drug guide, for instance. Then we'll look at using patient specific tables such as what you might find for a patient in an ICU or critical care transport situation. Finally, we'll look at some of the more popular tricks and shortcuts which I left until last on purpose. Later on we will talk about why they are at the very end of the book and have not appeared earlier.

Using pre-made tables is a very common method of determining drug doses and it is usually very safe, in most situations. When produced by a trusted resource such as a reputable publishing company or medical supply house, they are very reliable. They are commonly arranged by dose per weight so that you can merely reference a chart, find the patient's weight and then find the dose. Dosing on these charts is standardized to meet most but not all situations so some caution is still advised.

Tables and charts come in many shapes and sizes

depending on their source. It may be a photocopied dosing chart used by your unit in a hospital. It may be in the form of a drip rate table used in the back of a treatment protocol for EMS providers. Whatever the case, it is your job and responsibility as a health care professional to verify the source of the table or chart in order to determine its reliability. You should also be familiar enough with the approximate doses for a given drug so that you are not fooled by a typo in the table (they do happen).

Some pre-made tables are arranged for specific situations and caution should be used since some understanding of treatment context is important. For example, in the case of a pediatric ACLS dosing tape like the Broselow Tape, instead of dose per weight, they may be dose per height or length. In this case the tape is laid next to the child and where the child ends is where the dosing ranges start for that child. Because these are created for pediatric patients, this is one of those situations where understanding the treatment context is important. Doses for a very small adult who matches a range on the pediatric tape would not necessarily be appropriate.

The same is true for very obese patients whose dense muscle body weight is less than their total body weight and may cause overdosing on certain drugs. When in doubt, consult with the prescribing resource (physician, nurse practitioner, or PA) before using a standardized chart for these patients. Finally, there are pocket ACLS or EMS guides with dosing tables in them. The same rules for caution apply to these guides as well, but they can be a very valuable resource.

The reason I save this section for last is that you need to

have the basis for the formula to make the correct calculations on the fly. What if your pocket guide fell out during a motor vehicle extrication at an accident scene or someone used the last photocopied guide on your hospital unit and you need to dose your patient now? You need to know how to do the actual calculations. The use guides, charts and tables for getting your doses are just the icing on the med math cake, if you will.

Again, you must use caution! Avoid medication errors by knowing how to check your tables correctly.

What about patient specific tables?

Patient specific dosing tables are sometimes seen for inter-facility EMS transports by ambulance and I expect we'll see them more often since computers make creating these charts on a per patient basis easy. Since that is the case, it makes some sense to review patient specific tables and charts here. You may also see these created for specific patients in a critical care or intensive care unit setting.

Pediatric assessment tapes appear again here since they qualify as a patient specific table of a sort. Also, patients with chronic illnesses and medical needs may have tables for use in their home care situations where the caregivers may rotate in and out frequently. Special needs patients such as dialysis patients may have their own dosing regimen related to their specific limited kidney function.

To help with verifying whether a chart or table is appropriate for the patient, we can use something we all have learned along the way. I'll refer back to my early days as a basic EMT. For the rest of you, think of the five R's or five rights we covered earlier in the book. Ask yourself the question, "Is this chart for the right patient, right medication, right dose, or right dates?" If the patient has lost 40 pounds since the chart was made 2 months ago, it may not apply to them any more. That means you need to fall back on your formulas and med math.

In the case of specific patient orders, is there a physician's or nurse practitioner's signature accompanying the chart or table. This may not apply to every case but if it does, you should look for it.

Tips, Shortcuts and Tricks for Dosing

Let's move on to tips and tricks from the field. First off, this may or may not apply to nurses in a facility. You do not often have to guess a patient weight unless you are in the emergency department. You will likely have access to scales to weigh the patient and plenty of paper and calculators around. For the EMS providers and home care nurses, this will not always be the case, so I thought I would throw in a few pointers and tricks of the trade here.

First off, guessing a patient's weight can be a chore. Even though it would be nice to think of every adult as one hundred kilos or multiples thereof, you would end up under or overdosing many of your patients. Ask the patients themselves, family members, or even compare the unconscious patient to bystanders or members of your crew and ask them what they weigh. Careful with this one, though. You might end up offending some poor old lady watching you work.

Make sure you keep a pad of blank paper, pens, and a small calculator with you. Most smart phones have a calculator app on them now, so figure out how to access it for use when a situation arises. Medical control at the hospital or your home care nursing office can also be a resource. If you don't trust your calculations, don't guess. Have the doc at the hospital or another nurse back at the office give you a dose using the tables and resources at their fingertips.

Finally, for those using minidrip sets and not IV pumps, check your drip rates often and tape the roller valves down so they don't move as you transport the patient. Now let's move on to the old Paramedic's Tricks section.

I left this one for last on purpose because they really are cheating and should not be used without some caution. You can kill a patient if you are not very careful. I'm not exaggerating here. If you use these tips and methods, you do so at your own risk and the risk of your patient. They work in very specific situations only. Outside of those situations, they are worse than guessing. That said let's move on.

There are two primary methods used out there for two common paramedic drugs. The Dopamine and Lidocaine clocks and the Dopamine Divide by Ten (and subtract two) method. Let's start with the two clock methods.

Dopamine Clock Method

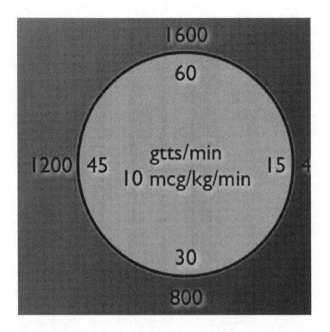

To do this method draw a circle. Inside the circle place 60 at the top of the circle, 15 at the 3 o'clock position, 30 at the 6 o'clock position, and 45 at the 9 o'clock position. Outside the circle place 1600 at the top of the circle, 400 at the 3 o'clock position, 800 at the 6 o'clock position, and 1200 at the 9 o'clock position. Now you are ready to see how this method works. This method works for multiples of 5 mcg/kg/min in a micro drip IV tubing set up (60 gtts/mL).

1) Multiply the patients weight in Kg x 10 (i.e., 80 x 10 = 800)

2) Find the 800 on the outside of the clock and the corresponding number on the inside of the clock will give

you the number of drops per minute (30 gtts/min) to equal 10 mcg/kg/min.

3) To give 5 mcg/kg/min just divide the inside number in half. To give 20 mcg/kg/min, double the inside number of drips.

4) Run the dopamine via either micro drip tubing, or, macro drip tubing with a Dial a Flow device.

The Rule of Fours Method (Lidocaine Clock Method)

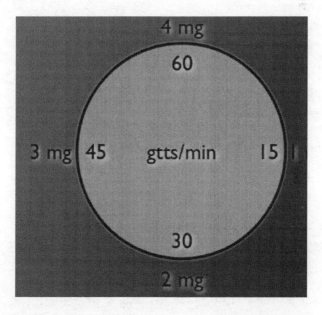

Start with some assumptions. (You know what that means) We assume that there are 4 mg of lidocaine for each milliliter of IV solution (That is, by putting 2 grams or 2000 mg of lidocaine into 500 ml of NS and dividing 2000 mg by 500 ml = 4 mg/ml). This means that there is 4 mg = 1 ml which means we will have 4mg for every 60 drops of solution because the drip set is a 60 gtts/ml IV set.

Use the same circle clock you drew in the Dopamine clock method. Keep the inside numbers corresponding to drip rates. On the outside put 4 mg at the 12 o'clock point, followed by 1 mg, 2 mg, and 3 mg each at the 3 o'clock, 6 o'clock and 9 o'clock respectively. For 1 mg of lidocaine per minute choose 15 gtts/min, for 2 mg of lidocaine per minute choose 30 gtts/min, and for 3 mg of lidocaine choose 45 gtts/min.

Dopamine 10 and 2 Method

This method assumes a patient who is 100 kg (220 lbs). Yes, it is another assumption method. Take that as another warning. Use this at your own (and your patient's) risk. Divide the patient's weight in pounds by 10, rounding down. (220 ÷ 10 = 22). Then you subtract 2 from that answer and that's close. By close, I mean that as patient's weights move farther from 100 kilos, this method becomes less accurate.

Ok, so you might be asking, "Jamie is there ever an appropriate time to use these shortcuts and tips from the old paramedic's back of tricks?" Sure there are. If you know that your instructor is looking for a real number on a test or practical testing situation then use the full math version. When the time comes to check your work, how do you do that? Use the corresponding trick for certain meds to see if you are in the ballpark or not.

For instance, the Dopamine ten and two method will

provide you with a check on the last dopamine problem we did in the earlier segment. A 220 pound man, divided by 10 and subtract two gives you a drip rate of 20. We came up with 19 so we are in the range and our number is probably correct. If we had used our initial finding of less than a drop per minute, we would know that we were wrong when double checking with this method.

Another time to use these shortcuts is in really unusual and urgent situations. In the case of a disaster situation I mean. This can be interpreted by the lawyers out there reading this as never. But, for the rest of you, if you find yourself in a situation when you literally have seconds to make a decision, make it and then make sure you come back and double check your dose correctly as soon as possible. Again, I can't recommend it but I will leave it up to you to decide when and where you might need these tricks.

Finally, in megacodes, instructors seem to love these things. It saves them time and for some it seems to show you "know the ropes." If you ever come by me in a megacode, though, you better do it the right way first! Then you can amaze me with your knowledge of parlor tricks and slight of hand.

Let's review:

- Use Pre-Made Tables Carefully
- Patient Specific Tables Are Useful
- Use Tricks and Shortcuts Sparingly

Remember, if you need more help there are additional resources and a complete video companion series and additional practice tests and quizzes for purchase to go with this book. It is available for those of you who might

Davis Jamie

need it at <u>MedMathSimplified.com/ebook</u>

PRACTICE QUIZ

1.) A client has an order for 20 g of Ampicillin. Ampicillin is available as 8,000 mg tablets. What should the nurse administer?

2.) A client is ordered for an infusion of 789 mL over the next 12.7 hr by infusion pump. What is the IV flow rate in mL/hr?

3.) A client is ordered Lasix 23 mg IV push now. Available: 10 mg in 10 mL. How much will the nurse draw up?

4.) A client is ordered 50 milligrams of Amitriptyline. 25 milligram tablets are available. How many tablets will you give?

5.) A client is ordered 37.5 milligrams of Nortriptyline. 25 milligram tablets are available. How many tablets will you give?

* * *

6.) A client is ordered 50 milligrams of Amoxicillin orally. 125 milligrams in 5 milliLiters (mL) of Syrup is available. How many milliLiters (mL) will you administer?

7.) A client is ordered 20 milligrams of Haloperidol by intramuscular injection. 50 milligrams in 1 milliLiter (mL) of liquid for IM Injection is available. How many milliLiters (mL) will you administer?

8.) A client is ordered 50 milligrams of Diphenhydramine intravenously. 250 milligrams in 10 milliLiters (mL) of liquid for IV Injection is available. How many milliLiters (mL) will you administer?

9.) A client is ordered 75 milligrams of Aminophylline intravenously. 250 milligrams in 10 milliLiters (mL) of liquid for IV Injection is available. How many milliLiters (mL) will you administer?

10.) A client is ordered 10 milligrams of Morphine by intramuscular injection. 5 milligrams in 1 milliLiter (mL) of liquid for IM Injection is the concentration on hand. How many milliLiters (mL) will you administer?

11.) A client is ordered 75 micrograms of Fentanyl intravenously. The concentration on hand is 0.1 milligrams in 1 milliLiter (mL) of liquid for IV Injection. How many milliLiters (mL) will you administer?

12.) A client is ordered 2.5 milligrams of Promethazine orally. 5 milligrams in 5 milliLiters (mL) of elixir is available. How many milliLiters (mL) will you administer?

* * *

13.) A client is ordered 0.25 g orally every 8 hours. How much will the nurse administer each dose if the available concentration is 125 mg per tablet?

14.) A client is ordered a dose of Zofran and 8 mg orally. There is a 100 milliLiter (mL) bottle of Zofran in a concentration of 4 mg per teaspoon. How many milliLiters (mL) will you give by mouth?

15.) A client is ordered a dose of Lactated Ringers (LR) IV fluid at the rate of 125 milliLiters (mL) per hour. How long will it take to infuse a 1 Liter bag of fluid in minutes?

Answers: 1.) 2.5 tablets of Ampicillin; 2.) 62.13 mL/hr; 3.) 23 mL of Lasix; 4.) 2 tablets; 5.) 1.5 tablets; 6.) 2 milliLiters (mL); 7.) 0.4 milliLiters (mL); 8.) 2 milliLiter (mL); 9.) 3 milliLiter (mL); 10.) 2 milliLiters (mL); 11.) 0.75 milliLiters (mL); 12.) 2.5 milliLiters (mL); 13.) 2 tablets; 14.) 10 milliLiters (mL); 15.) 480 minutes (8 hours).

ADDITIONAL RESOURCES

Want More?

You can get more Med Math Practice and receive updates on other titles from Jamie Davis, "the Podmedic." Visit www.medmathsimplified.com/ebook and sign up for the special Med Math Email List which will give you access to additional resources and updates from Jamie's shows online.

Did you like the book? Help others find it so they can master med math. Please leave an honest review of the book at Amazon.com.

About the Author

Jamie Davis, RN, NRP, B.A., A.S., host of the Nursing Show is a nationally recognized medical educator who began educating new emergency responders as a training officer for his local EMS program. As a media producer, he has been recognized for the MedicCast Podcast, a weekly program for emergency medical providers like EMTs and paramedics, and the Nursing Show, a similar program for nurses and nursing students. His programs and resources have been downloaded over 4 million times by listeners and viewers.

Jamie speaks nationally on health care, technology, and education and is an advocate for integrating podcasting and media creation in schools at all levels. He has spoken at the Podcast and New Media Expo, been a featured faculty member of the Podcast Secrets course, and has been invited to speak and MC at medical conferences and expos around the world.

Jamie is also the managing director of the ProMed Network, a collection of the best and brightest independent medical podcasters and new media creators currently available online. The network now comprises over 30 independently produced programs for medical and health care professionals at all levels. These trusted resources for high quality medical education and information reach over 500,000 downloads to medical professionals every month.

Made in the USA
Middletown, DE
27 May 2016